I0209834

40 Juice Recipe Solutions to Your Overweight Problems:

Quickly and Naturally Burn Fat Fast to Look Your Best in No Time!

By

Joe Correa CSN

COPYRIGHT

© 2017 Live Stronger Faster Inc.

All rights reserved

Reproduction or translation of any part of this work beyond that permitted by section 107 or 108 of the 1976 United States Copyright Act without the permission of the copyright owner is unlawful.

This publication is designed to provide accurate and authoritative information in regard to the subject matter covered. It is sold with the understanding that neither the author nor the publisher is engaged in rendering medical advice. If medical advice or assistance is needed, consult with a doctor. This book is considered a guide and should not be used in any way detrimental to your health. Consult with a physician before starting this nutritional plan to make sure it's right for you.

ACKNOWLEDGEMENTS

This book is dedicated to my friends and family that have had mild or serious illnesses so that you may find a solution and make the necessary changes in your life.

40 Juice Recipe Solutions to Your Overweight Problems:

Quickly and Naturally Burn Fat Fast to Look Your Best in No Time!

By

Joe Correa CSN

CONTENTS

ABOUT THE AUTHOR

After years of Research, I honestly believe in the positive effects that proper nutrition can have over the body and mind. My knowledge and experience has helped me live healthier throughout the years and which I have shared with family and friends. The more you know about eating and drinking healthier, the sooner you will want to change your life and eating habits.

Nutrition is a key part in the process of being healthy and living longer so get started today. The first step is the most important and the most significant.

INTRODUCTION

40 Juice Recipe Solutions to Your Overweight Problems: Quickly and Naturally Burn Fat Fast to Look Your Best in No Time!

By Joe Correa CSN

Staying fit and healthy has become a number one priority in life for most people. The goal for you should be to have good nutrition and a weight loss plan.

Combining a proper diet with a well-organized physical activity and a complete body detox has been recognized to be the most effective way to achieve your goal of loosing those extra pounds.

Unfortunately, we often don't seem to have enough time for cooking and preparing meals which means we aren't getting the nutrients we need. Besides that, having a proper detox plan is necessary for weight loss and this is almost impossible without implementing juices in your diet. This is why most nutritionists agree that juicing is the number one option for weight loss and a complete body detoxification.

First, let's go over some of the benefits juicing has in general. If you're not the type of person who enjoys eating fruits and veggies throughout the day, juicing can get you large amounts of nutrients and minerals in just one drink. A simple kale, carrot, ginger, parsley, and apple juice with your lunch will taste amazing and give you enough of the necessary nutrients you need. Even better, replace your breakfast or dinner with one of these nutrient-rich power juices, and your weight loss results will be inevitable.

The bottom line is, YOU CAN rely on juicing as your sole source of fruits and veggies per day. Getting the nutrients you need through juices is the most convenient way to lose weight!

These amazing juice recipes focus on getting you the weight loss results in the healthiest way possible. You can forget those impossible diets and extreme nutrition regimes. Juices full of healthy fruits and vegetables will speed up your metabolism, give you plenty of vitamins and minerals, improve your overall health, and burn those nasty fats fast. Improving your well being in general will make you more fit, active, and will reduce the risk of many different diseases. These weight loss juice recipes will make a significant change in your life, health and future.

40 JUICE RECIPE SOLUTIONS TO YOUR OVERWEIGHT PROBLEMS: QUICKLY AND NATURALLY BURN FAT FAST TO LOOK YOUR BEST IN NO TIME!

1.   Fresh Lime Detox Juice

Ingredients:

2 large cucumbers, peeled

2 large limes, peeled

1 cup of beet greens, torn

1 cup of kale, chopped

1 cup of parsley, chopped

1 tbsp of agave syrup

½ cup of pure coconut water, unsweetened

Preparation:

Wash and prepare the ingredients.

Run through a juicer, one at the time. Combine with unsweetened coconut water and add one tablespoon of agave syrup. Mix well and serve cold.

Nutritional information per serving: Kcal: 139, Protein: 10.6g, Carbs: 42.2g, Fats: 1.9g

2. Tomato Juice

Ingredients:

3 large tomatoes

2 large carrots, sliced

2 celery stalks

1 large cucumber

1 bunch of fresh spinach

1 large bell pepper

Preparation:

Wash and prepare the ingredients. Combine all ingredients in a juicer and process until juiced. Transfer to a serving glasses and serve, or refrigerate before use. Sprinkle with some fresh mint, but this is optional.

Nutritional information per serving: Kcal: 248, Protein: 3.71g, Carbs: 70.5g, Fats: 3.71g

3.   Beet Pear Juice

Ingredients:

1 medium-sized beet, trimmed

1 large lemon, peeled

3 large pears

1 cup of fresh raspberries

Preparation:

Combine all ingredients in a juicer or a blender. Process until nicely smooth and transfer to a serving glass. Add few ice cubes before serving or refrigerate until use.

Nutritional information per serving: Kcal: 378, Protein: 2.7g, Carbs: 133g, Fats: 2.7g

4.   Chia Pepper Juice

Ingredients:

3 tbsp of chia seeds

1 large lemon, peeled

½ red bell pepper, seeded

½ yellow bell pepper, seeded

1 green apple, cored

Preparation:

Wash and prepare the ingredients. Run all except chia seeds trough the juicer. Stir in the chia seeds and set aside for 15 minutes before use.

Nutritional information per serving: Kcal: 136, Protein: 4.3g, Carbs: 31.2g, Fats: 6.1g

5.　　Apricot Grapefruit Juice

Ingredients:

1 large apricot, pitted

1 large grapefruit, peeled

1 cup of broccoli

1 large banana

Preparation:

Wash the ingredients and run trough a juicer. Add few ice cubes or refrigerate for 30 minutes before serving.

Nutritional information per serving: Kcal: 229, Protein: 6.5g, Carbs: 67.2g, Fats: 1.3g

6.   Ginger Butternut Squash Juice

Ingredients:

½ cup of butternut squash cubes

2 slices of fresh ginger

1 large red delicious apple, peeled and cored

1 large carrot

1 tbsp of fresh mint, finely chopped

1 large orange, peeled

1 tsp of pure coconut sugar

Preparation:

Run the ingredients through a juicer.

Transfer to a serving glass and stir in one teaspoon of pure coconut sugar.

Serve with ice.

Nutritional information per serving: Kcal: 314, Protein: 5.3g, Carbs: 61g, Fats: 1.2g

7.   Honeydew Melon Juice

Ingredients:

2 large honeydew melon wedges

5 tbsp of fresh mint

1 cup of avocado, peeled and pitted

1 large lime, peeled

Preparation:

Combine all ingredients in a juicer and process until juiced.

Transfer to serving glasses and add few ice cubes. Enjoy!

Nutritional information per serving: Kcal: 321, Protein: 5.2g, Carbs: 46.8g, Fats: 22.6g

8.   Berry Beet Juice

Ingredients:

1 cup of blackberries

1 cup of blueberries

1 cup of fresh basil

1 large beet, trimmed

2 oz of coconut water

Preparation:

Wash and prepare the fruits and vegetables.

Run trough the juicer and stir in the coconut water. Add few ice cubes and serve immediately.

Nutritional information per serving: Kcal: 142, Protein: 5.2g, Carbs: 44.8g, Fats: 1.5g

9.   Pomegranate Watermelon Juice

Ingredients:

1 cup of watermelon, peeled and seeded

1 large orange, peeled

1 cup of Romaine lettuce, shredded

1 cup of pomegranate seeds

Preparation:

Wash and prepare the ingredients. Run trough the juicer and refrigerate before use.

Nutritional information per serving: Kcal: 142, Protein: 5.2g, Carbs: 44.8g, Fats: 1.5g

10.   Asparagus-Olive Oil Juice

Ingredients:

1 large green apple, cored

4 medium-sized asparagus spears, trimmed

1 large broccoli

3 large celery stalks

1 tbsp of extra-virgin olive oil

A handful of fresh parsley

Preparation:

Combine apple, asparagus, broccoli, and celery in a juicer and process until juiced.

Transfer to serving glasses and stir in the olive oil. Refrigerate for 1 hour before serving. Garnish with some fresh parsley.

Nutritional information per serving: Kcal: 234, Protein: 7.3g, Carbs: 45.9g, Fats: 10.7g

11.   Green Kiwi Juice

Ingredients:

2 whole leeks, chopped

1 cup of Brussel sprouts, chopped

1 cup of parsley, chopped

2 whole kiwis, chopped

A handful of spinach, chopped

½ cup of water

Preparation:

Run the ingredients through a juicer.

Serve cold.

Nutritional information per serving: Kcal: 207, Protein: 9.8g, Carbs: 58.1g, Fats: 2.1g

12. Summer Guava Juice

Ingredients:

1 cup of pineapple chunks

1 whole guava, chopped

2 cups of chard, chopped

2 whole lemons, peeled

½ cup of coconut water, unsweetened

Preparation:

Run the ingredients through a juicer, one at the time.

Add coconut water and mix well.

Serve immediately.

Nutritional information per serving: Kcal: 130, Protein: 4.8g, Carbs: 43g, Fats: 1.2g

13.   Turnip Artichoke Juice

Ingredients:

1 cup of turnip greens

1 large cucumber

1 large artichoke head

5 large asparagus spears

Preparation:

Combine all ingredients in a juicer and process until juiced.

Transfer to serving glasses and add few ice cubes before serving.

Nutritional information per serving: Kcal: 101, Protein: 10.1g, Carbs: 35.8g, Fats: 0.8g

14.   Grapefruit Kiwi Juice

Ingredients:

2 kiwis, peeled

1 cup of carrots, chopped

2 cups of green cabbage, shredded

1 whole grapefruit, peeled

1 tbsp of honey, raw

Preparation:

Run the ingredients through a juicer.

Add one tablespoon of honey and serve immediately.

Nutritional information per serving: Kcal: 219, Protein: 6.9g, Carbs: 69g, Fats: 1.5g

15.   Cherry Juice

Ingredients:

1 cup of cherries, pitted

1 medium-sized banana

1 large cucumber

1 large carrot

Preparation:

Wash the cherries, cucumber, and carrot. Run all trough the juicer and add few ice cubes.

Serve immediately.

Nutritional information per serving: Kcal: 238, Protein: 5.5g, Carbs: 69.4g, Fats: 1.2g

16. Bell Pepper Juice

Ingredients:

1 small red bell pepper, seeded

1 small green bell pepper, seeded

1 small yellow bell pepper, seeded

1 cup of broccoli

1 cup of fresh kale

Preparation:

Wash and prepare the vegetables.

Process in a juicer and refrigerate for 1 hour before serving. Sprinkle with some Cayenne pepper if you like it spicier. However, this is optional.

Nutritional information per serving: Kcal: 114, Protein: 8.7g, Carbs: 31.5g, Fats: 1.7g

17.   Fennel Brussel Sprouts Juice

Ingredients:

1 large fennel bulb

1 cup of Brussel Sprouts

2 large leeks

½ tsp of fresh rosemary

Preparation:

Combine all ingredients in a juicer and process until juiced.

Transfer to a serving glass and add few ice cubes, or refrigerate before serving.

Nutritional information per serving: Kcal: 165, Protein: 8.5g, Carbs: 50.1g, Fats: 1.3g

18. Turnip Greens and Cranberry Juice

Ingredients:

1 cup of turnip greens, chopped

1 cup of cranberries

1 cup of baby spinach, torn

1 whole lemon, peeled

½ cup of pure coconut water

Preparation:

Juice the ingredients and combine with coconut water.

Serve with ice.

Nutritional information per serving: Kcal: 69, Protein: 4.3g, Carbs: 27.6g, Fats: 0.8g

19. Zucchini Watercress Juice

Ingredients:

1 medium-sized zucchini

1 cup of watercress

3 large carrots

1 tbsp of fresh parsley

Preparation:

Wash and prepare the ingredients.

Run trough the juicer and add some ice before serving.

Nutritional information per serving: Kcal: 165, Protein: 8.5g, Carbs: 50.1g, Fats: 1.3g

20.　Parsnip Peach Juice

Ingredients:

1 large peach, peeled

1 cup of parsnip, sliced

1 small orange, peeled

3 cups of red leaf lettuce, torn

1 tsp of agave syrup

Preparation:

Juice the ingredients and add one teaspoon of agave syrup

Mix well and serve immediately.

Nutritional information per serving: Kcal: 177, Protein: 5.2g, Carbs: 53.7g, Fats: 1.1g

21.   Guava Mango Juice

Ingredients:

1 large guava, peeled

1 large mango

1 large lime, peeled

3 oz of coconut water

Preparation:

Wash the fruits and peel the lime. Process in a juicer and transfer to serving glasses.

Add coconut water and stir well.

Refrigerate for 1 hour before serving.

Nutritional information per serving: Kcal: 225, Protein: 4.4g, Carbs: 63.9g, Fats: 1.8g

22.   Fresh Grape Juice

Ingredients:

2 cups of grapes

1 cup of kale, chopped

1 whole grapefruit, peeled

1 cup of watercress, chopped

½ cup of water

Preparation:

Run the ingredients through a juicer.

Serve immediately.

Nutritional information per serving: Kcal: 231, Protein: 6.7g, Carbs: 64g, Fats: 1.6g

23.   Tomato Basil Juice

Ingredients:

1 large tomato

1 cup of fresh basil

1 large cucumber

½ tsp of fresh rosemary

Preparation:

Combine all ingredients in a juicer and process until juiced.

Transfer to serving glasses and serve immediately.

Nutritional information per serving: Kcal: 67, Protein: 4.3g, Carbs: 18.6g, Fats: 0.8g

24.   Sweet Potato Radish Juice

Ingredients:

1 cup of red leaf lettuce

1 small radish, trimmed

1 large zucchini

1 medium-sized sweet potato, peeled

1 tsp of ginger root

Preparation:

Wash and prepare the ingredients. Combine all in a juicer and process until juiced.

Transfer to serving glasses and serve immediately.

Nutritional information per serving: Kcal: 67, Protein: 4.3g, Carbs: 18.6g, Fats: 0.8g

25.   Kiwi Pineapple Juice

Ingredients:

3 large kiwis, peeled

1 cup of pineapple chunks, cubed

1 medium-sized orange, peeled

1 cup of beet greens, trimmed

1 tbsp of fresh mint

Preparation:

Wash and prepare all ingredients. Run all ingredients trough a juicer, one at a time.

Add few ice cubes and serve immediately.

Nutritional information per serving: Kcal: 228, Protein: 5.4g, Carbs: 69.3g, Fats: 1.5g

26.   Orange Pumpkin Juice

Ingredients:

1 cup of pumpkin, seeded and peeled

1 large orange, peeled

1 cup of purple cabbage

1 large green apple, cored

1 tsp of ginger root

Preparation:

Wash and prepare the ingredients. Combine all in a juicer and process until juiced.

Refrigerate for 30 minutes before serving.

Nutritional information per serving: Kcal: 228, Protein: 5.4g, Carbs: 69.3g, Fats: 1.5g

27.   Papaya Strawberry Juice

Ingredients:

1 small papaya, seeded and peeled

1 large lime, peeled

1 cup of strawberries

1 cup of cranberries

3 oz of coconut water

Preparation:

Wash and prepare all ingredients. Combine papaya, lime, strawberries, and cranberries in a juicer. Process until juiced.

Stir in the coconut water and refrigerate for 30 minutes before serving.

Nutritional information per serving: Kcal: 153, Protein: 2.6g, Carbs: 50.9g, Fats: 1.8g

28.   Avocado Cantaloupe Juice

Ingredients:

1 cup of avocado, peeled and pitted

1 cup of cantaloupe, peeled and chopped

1 large cucumber

1 large lemon, peeled

Preparation:

Combine all ingredients in a juicer and process until juiced. Transfer to serving glasses and add few ice cubes.

Serve immediately.

Nutritional information per serving: Kcal: 292, Protein: 6.8g, Carbs: 41.5g, Fats: 22.2g

29.   Ginger Blueberry Juice

Ingredients:

2 slices of ginger, fresh

1 cup of collard greens, chopped

1 cup of blueberries, fresh

1 cup of pomegranate seeds

1 whole lime

1 cup of turnip greens, chopped

1 tbsp of honey, raw

Preparation:

Juice the ingredients and add one tablespoon of honey.

Mix well and serve.

Nutritional information per serving: Kcal: 159, Protein: 4.7g, Carbs: 48g, Fats: 1.9g

30. Plum Peach Juice

Ingredients:

5 large plums, pitted

2 large peaches, pitted

1 cup of pomegranate seeds

1 large carrot

Preparation:

Wash and prepare the ingredients. Run trough the juicer, one at a time.

Refrigerate for 30 minutes before serving.

Nutritional information per serving: Kcal: 326, Protein: 7.6g, Carbs: 94.2g, Fats: 3.1g

31. Swiss Chard Kale Juice

Ingredients:

1 cup of Swiss chard

1 cup of fresh kale

1 cup of Romaine lettuce

1 large tomato

1 large fennel bulb

1 cup of collard greens

Preparation:

Wash and prepare all ingredients. Run trough the juicer, one at a time.

Serve immediately or refrigerate for 20 minutes before use.

Nutritional information per serving: Kcal: 106, Protein: 9.7g, Carbs: 34.8g, Fats: 1.8g

32. Cantaloupe Juice

Ingredients:

1 cup of cantaloupe, diced

1 cup of beet greens

1 medium-sized radish, chopped

1 tbsp of fresh mint, chopped

1 cup of cauliflower, chopped

Preparation:

Run the ingredients through a juicer.

Serve immediately with some ice.

Nutritional information per serving: Kcal: 123, Protein: 8.1g, Carbs: 37.7g, Fats: 1.1g

33.   Blueberry Pear Juice

Ingredients:

2 large pears, peeled and seeds removed

1 cup of blueberries, fresh

1 medium-sized radish, sliced

1 tbsp of fresh mint, chopped

1 cup of cauliflower, chopped

¼ cup of coconut water, unsweetened

Preparation:

Wash and prepare the ingredients.

Run through a juicer and combine with coconut water.

Serve immediately.

Nutritional information per serving: Kcal: 297, Protein: 4.9g, Carbs: 97g, Fats: 1.4g

34.   Tomato Cleaning Juice

Ingredients:

2 large tomatoes, peeled

1 cup of beets, chopped

1 cup of fennel, sliced

1 tbsp of fresh mint, chopped

1 cup of red leaf lettuce, shredded

½ tsp of ginger, ground

Preparation:

Juice the ingredients and combine with ground ginger.

Serve cold.

Nutritional information per serving: Kcal: 111, Protein: 6.9g, Carbs: 34.8g, Fats: 1.2g

35.   Wild Berry Juice

Ingredients:

1 cup of raspberries, fresh

1 cup of blackberries, fresh

1 cup of blueberries, fresh

2 slices od ginger

½ cup of pure coconut water, unsweetened

Preparation:

Wash and drain the berries. Run through a juicer and combine with coconut water.

Serve cold.

Nutritional information per serving: Kcal: 176, Protein: 3.7g, Carbs: 58.3g, Fats: 1.8g

36.   Mustard Greens Apple Juice

Ingredients:

1 cup of mustard greens, chopped

1 granny smith apple, peeled and cored

1 large artichoke, chopped

1 cup of Brussel sprouts

½ tsp of cinnamon, freshly ground

½ cup of pure coconut water, unsweetened

1 tsp of agave nectar

Preparation:

Prepare the ingredients and run through a juicer.

Transfer to a serving glass and combine with unsweetened coconut water. Add one teaspoon of agave nectar and some cinnamon to taste.

Serve immediately.

Nutritional information per serving: Kcal: 195, Protein: 13.7g, Carbs: 63.4g, Fats: 1.3g

37.   Artichoke Cabbage Juice

Ingredients:

1 medium-sized artichoke head

1 cup of green cabbage

1 large cucumber

1 large lemon, peeled

A handful of spinach

Preparation:

Wash and prepare the ingredients. Run trough the juicer, on at a time.

Transfer to serving glasses and add few ice cubes before serving.

Nutritional information per serving: Kcal: 99, Protein: 8.8g, Carbs: 36.4g, Fats: 0.9g

38. Grape Radish Juice

Ingredients:

2 large carrots

3 large radishes, trimmed

1 large orange, peeled

1 cup of green grapes

1 tsp of ginger root, grated

Preparation:

Wash and prepare the ingredients. Combine carrots, radishes, orange, and grapes in a juicer. Process until juiced.

Transfer to serving glasses and add few ice cubes or refrigerate before serving.

Nutritional information per serving: Kcal: 176, Protein: 3.9g, Carbs: 52.5g, Fats: 0.9g

39.   Parsnip Beet Juice

Ingredients:

1 cup of parsnip, chopped

1 cup of beets, trimmed

1 cup of beet greens, trimmed

1 small cauliflower head

2 tbsp of fresh parsley

Preparation:

Wash and prepare the ingredients. Run trough a juicer and transfer to serving glasses.

Add few ice cubes and serve or refrigerate for 20 minutes before serving.

Enjoy!

Nutritional information per serving: Kcal: 166, Protein: 9.9g, Carbs: 52.3g, Fats: 1.5g

40.   Spicy Tomato Juice

Ingredients:

1 cup of cherry tomatoes

1 medium-sized spring onion

1 large bell pepper, seeded

1 garlic clove, peeled

¼ tsp of Cayenne pepper, ground

¼ tsp of salt

A handful of fresh cilantro

Preparation:

Wash and prepare the vegetables. Combine tomatoes, spring onion, bell pepper, and garlic in a juicer. Process until juiced and transfer to serving glasses. Stir in the salt and Cayenne pepper.

Serve immediately.

Nutritional information per serving: Kcal: 41, Protein: 2.8g, Carbs: 11.5g, Fats: 0.6g

ADDITIONAL TITLES FROM THIS AUTHOR

70 Effective Meal Recipes to Prevent and Solve Being Overweight: Burn Fat Fast by Using Proper Dieting and Smart Nutrition

By

Joe Correa CSN

48 Acne Solving Meal Recipes: The Fast and Natural Path to Fixing Your Acne Problems in Less Than 10 Days!

By

Joe Correa CSN

41 Alzheimer's Preventing Meal Recipes: Reduce or Eliminate Your Alzheimer's Condition in 30 Days or Less!

By

Joe Correa CSN

70 Effective Breast Cancer Meal Recipes: Prevent and Fight Breast Cancer with Smart Nutrition and Powerful Foods

By

Joe Correa CSN

www.ingramcontent.com/pod-product-compliance
Lightning Source LLC
Chambersburg PA
CBHW051040030426
42336CB00015B/2964